Turmeric: A Cancer Cure?

The Amazing Health and Beauty Benefits of Turmeric

By Ryder Management Inc.

ISBN: 13:978-1503376755
ISBN: 10:1503376753
ASIN: B00ICCIINO

FORWARD

"Let food be thy medicine and medicine be thy food."
Hippocrates

.

Table of Contents

Preface

After refusing any form of the "cut, poison and burn" method of cancer treatment, I began an extensive on-line search for another way. My thoughts were to start in India and China since their medicine (both TCM and Ayurveda) predates that of North America.

This research led me to "turmeric" and its effective use in Ayurveda, a system of medicine practiced in India for over four thousand years.

Although I was not familiar with turmeric nor Ayurveda at the time, the more I learned about turmeric, the more fascinated I became and ultimately ordered organic turmeric supplements, from a supplier in India.

Wanting to know as much as I could about this plant, I continued studying all the information I could locate on turmeric. What puzzled me however, despite the large amount of studies and reports available on the effectiveness of turmeric, both on-line and in print, Canada and US health sources continue to state "lack of reliable evidence exist to support the use of turmeric for any health condition because few clinical trials have been conducted." My first thought upon reading this, included – Is North America healthcare really that far behind in their research concerning viable remedies?

Since I began studying turmeric well over three years ago, its reported benefits continue to increase, and includes posted testimony regarding its efficacy.

Curcumin, the main active constituent in turmeric, is nothing short of amazing! This book shares current information describing the many benefits turmeric has to offer from regular use. In addition, there are recipes for both health and beauty that are tried and true as being effective in the stated application and use.

Introduction

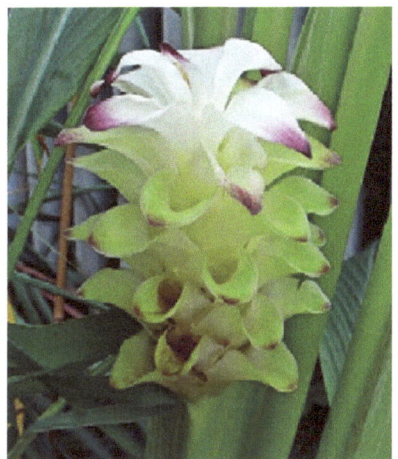

Flower of the Turmeric Plant

Turmeric is one of the most widely used spices around the world and is a great source of many health and beauty benefits. Turmeric (Curcuma longa) is a *rhizomatous herbaceous perennial* plant of the ginger family, **Zingiberaceae**. It is native to the tropical regions of south and southeastern Asia requiring temperatures between 20 C and 30 C to grow and requiring a considerable amount of rainfall to thrive. This leafy "stem-less" perennial has oblong shaped miniature scented leaves with rather long pale white spike-like flower clusters and it typically grows up to a meter in height. As a spice, yellow rhizomatous roots characterize turmeric. The spice we know as turmeric is obtained from these roots, similar to ginger. Removing the outer brown layer from the root reveals an orange-yellow or golden inside flesh. The taste of turmeric has been described as light and very mild with just a hint of orange and ginger along with a mild peppery taste.

India is the largest producer of turmeric followed by Thailand, Central America, Latin America and Taiwan. United Arab Emirates (UAE) is the largest importer of Indian turmeric.

General Uses

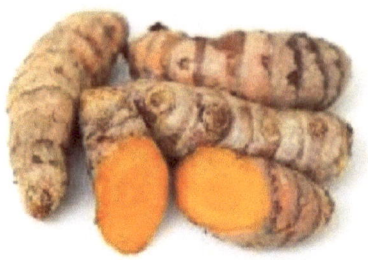

Turmeric root

Turmeric roots and leaves have a long history of use in traditional Indian and Chinese cuisine. Although turmeric may resemble ginger in appearance, its distinctive -yellow-orange flesh sets it apart. Despite turmeric's extensive use in the kitchen, it has voluminous benefits for the human body and a long history of use in both Ayurveda and TCM, two of the world's oldest systems of medicine.

Turmeric has been used in food preservation and is also a natural dye for textiles, where it is known as *food coloring E100*. Curcumin, a polyphenol compound of turmeric, is what gives rise to its orange - yellow color. Curcumin was first isolated and identified over two hundred years ago. Since 1900 BC, the beginning of Ayurveda medicine in India, various therapeutic methods have been assigned to turmeric in the treatment of a host of conditions. Turmeric's use includes conditions associated with the skin, heart, gut, liver, brain and wound healing.

Curcumin has been studied extensively for its ability to exhibit antioxidant, anti-inflammatory, antiviral, antibacterial, antifungal, anti-ulcer, anti-platelet, anti-scabies, anti-depressant and anticancer activities. Consequently turmeric has the potential to ward off a great many serious diseases including, but not limited to cancer, heart disease, liver disease and Alzheimer's.

Dr. Mercola, in commenting on the above, writes "…curcumin changes the regulation of DNA to help kill cancer."

Turmeric, known as "Haldi", "Haldee" or "Holud" in the Indian subcontinent, is also known as Indian Saffron, Zirsood, Turmeric, Olena and Terre-Merite in other parts of the world.

Chemical and Nutritional Value

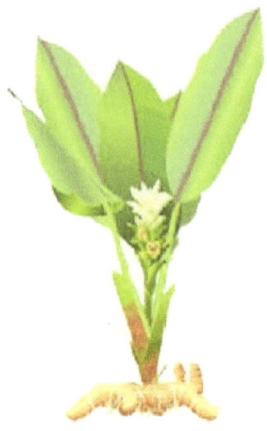

Turmeric art

The most important chemical compounds found in curcumin are a group called **curcuminoids**. Curcuminoids are a linear diarylheptanoids – also known as diphenylheptanoids – a small class of secondary metabolites whose molecules include curcumin and other derivatives. These natural polyphenols improve cell communication and reduce inflammation.

Other phytochemicals in turmeric include health benefitting volatile essential oils (called terpenes) such as termerone, zingiberene, and p-tolymehyl. Other terpenes include Alpha-pinene, alpha-terpineol, azulene, beta-carotene, borneol, caffeic acid, caryophyllene, cinnamic acid, eugenol, guaicol, limonene, linalool, p-coumaric acid, p-cymene, turmerone, vanillic acid, phellandrene, sabinene, curlone, curumene, cineole along with demethoxycurcumin, bisdemethoxycurcumin, and so many more. Each has many health benefits alone but also provide unique synergistic benefits too.

Turmeric also has notable phyto-nutrients and contains one of the highest anti-oxidant strengths known in the herb and spice world. Essential vitamins and minerals that are found in high quantity in turmeric include: vitamin C; vitamins B1, B2, B3; A and E. Minerals include calcium, chromium, iron, manganese, phosphorous, potassium, selenium and zinc. Several carotenoids, xanthrophyllis and carotenes convert to vitamin A as needed by the body for immunity purposes or they combat free radicals and, according to the Mayo Clinic, prevent heart disease.

As an example of the high quantity of nutrients found in turmeric, note the following example:

One tablespoon of powdered turmeric contains the following Recommended Daily Allowance (RDA) of vitamins and minerals:

Iron = 80%; vitamin B-6 = 21%; niacin = 5%; vitamin C = 7%; vitamin E = 3%; potassium = 8%; zinc = 6%; dietary fiber = 8% and cholesterol= 0%.

Curcumin also helps to control blood LDL or "bad cholesterol" levels. A small amount of turmeric per day either in the form of powder, crushed root or fresh root, is able to provide enough nutrients to help prevent many health conditions such as memory disorders, many types of cancers, infectious diseases, high blood pressure, strokes, respiratory disease, and heart disease .

Adverse reactions associated with turmeric have been reported in a small number of individuals when their dose exceeded eight grams per day for an extended period of use in excess of four months. These adverse effects were reported to be nausea and diarrhea. At the time of this writing, and considering that turmeric has been used medicinally in Ayurveda medicine for thousands of years, there is no scientific proof that turmeric has any real known side effects that can be considered negative.

Turmeric for Beauty

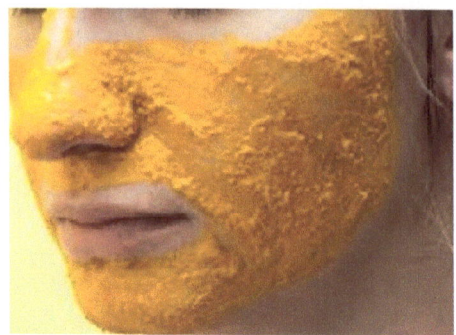

Turmeric face mask

Turmeric is widely used in the beauty industry in the Indian subcontinent. Many beauty products are made with turmeric as the main ingredient. Turmeric is also known as "Haldi" or "Holud" in the Indian subcontinent. Examples of turmeric's use in beauty treatments include:

As a treatment for acne and other skin conditions such as boils, blackheads, dry or oily skin; removal of dark circles, wrinkles and facial hair; smooth skin pigmentation; treatment for sunburns; effective for certain hair conditions including hair loss. These and other conditions can be resolved with the use of turmeric. Turmeric can be made into a paste by adding water, lemon juice, milk or coconut oil in a quantity (a few drops or more) large enough to make a paste. More specific beauty recipes made with turmeric are included at the end of this book.

Specific use in beauty routines:

Antibiotic and antiseptic properties both work against acne. Acne scars and inflammation are reduced with the regular use of a turmeric facemask (simple mixture of turmeric and lemon juice). Leave on face for 15 minutes, before rinsing off with warm water.

Turmeric powder mixed with buttermilk to form a paste can be applied to the eye, face and neck area for approximately twenty minutes a day to help treat wrinkles, rosacea along with dark circles under the eyes.

Cracked heels are bad to look at. Turmeric works as a good healing product. A few drops of coconut oil added to 3 tablespoons of turmeric powder can offer immediate relief to cracked heels. This mixture will also help prevent fungal infections that can arise between toes (often called athlete's foot).

Turmeric mixed with a few grams of flour and water can remove the dead cells from the skin and improve the skins elasticity.

Turmeric for scalp health – mixing turmeric with olive oil applied to the scalp for fifteen minutes before washing out with a natural shampoo can treat dandruff and other scalp issues. This formula can also be used to promote hair growth.

A paste made with turmeric and honey can be applied to the face and neck as a method of exfoliation. This simple paste will also help keep a check on pores.

Turmeric is also used as a teeth whitener.

The antiseptic properties found in turmeric can offer quick relief to burns and assist in more rapid healing.

Chickpea flour (sattu) or gram flour added to kasturi turmeric can be used as a facial scrub to inhibit hair growth. Be sure to apply this paste for about a month in order to notice results.

Since regular turmeric can temporarily stain the skin, "kasturi" turmeric (curcuma aromatica) is non-staining yet retains the acne clearing properties. This type of turmeric is not edible and therefore should only be used externally. Gram flour, also known as besan flour, chickpea flour or garbanzo flour is also used in homemade recipes with turmeric to cleanse and exfoliate the face.

Turmeric as Medicine

Although turmeric has been in use for thousands of years, certain claims exist that indicate there is not enough scientific evidence to support any health claims associated with turmeric's use. Despite this, a multitude of evidence does in fact exist to support the beneficial and medicinal use of turmeric (PubMed for example). In addition, a number of people can vouch for the efficacy of turmeric in all that it is purported to do.

Turmeric is available in North America in capsule form and used as a health supplement. In this method of delivery in India, it is referred to as "Holy powder".

Following are examples of turmeric's use in current medicine (from PubMed.gov unless otherwise indicated):

Turmeric is used in the treatment of arthritis, eczema, psoriasis, heartburn, ulcers, gallstones, kidney stones and anemia.

Turmeric can reduce the chances of prostate cancer when used regularly and this can be further enhanced when combined as a topping on cauliflower.

Turmeric also reduces the risk of many other forms of cancer and is considered in new anticancer drug development. According to the *American Association of Pharmaceutical Scientists*, turmeric has been successfully used as a treatment for colorectal cancer, pancreatic cancer, breast cancer, liver cancer and multiple myeloma. Reports show that curcumin can influence many cell-signaling pathways involved in tumor initiation and proliferation.

Improve overall mood – turmeric has been shown to enhance brain chemicals such as noradrenalin and serotonin and increases the production of dopamine, which determines how we experience pleasure and pain. A 2011 study published in the journal *Acta Poloniae Pharmaceutica* found that curcumin acted in the same way as the antidepressants Prozac and Imipramine do. In fact, a new study published in the journal of *Phytotherapy Research* has confirmed that turmeric is both safe and effective in treating serious states of depression.

Turmeric's anti-inflammatory properties reduce arthritis and rheumatoid arthritis flare-ups; and regular use of this spice has the ability to reduce overall body and bone aches and pains.

Turmeric increases the brain's kinetic energy, reducing the risk of Alzheimer's. Studies have shown unique bonding characteristics within turmeric, make it easier to penetrate the blood-brain barrier and bind with amyloid beta (Abeta). Abeta accumulation in the brain cells combined with oxidative stress and inflammation causes Alzheimer disease.

Turmeric is effective in cardiovascular respiratory health.

Turmeric purifies the bloodstream and reduces menstrual pain.

Turmeric stimulates the gallbladder to produce bile, which in turn, improves digestion and reduces bloating and gas.

Turmeric is a cost effective method in the treatment of irritable bowel syndrome and celiac disease.

A study published in the Fundamental U Clinical Pharmacology journal revealed that curcumin is effective in reversing and preventing cirrhosis of the liver.

Turmeric is also a natural and effective great pesticide. Sprinkle turmeric powder at all entry points to ward off insects, ants and termites.

Dr. Mercola has stated that turmeric is five to eight times stronger than vitamin E and stronger than vitamin C and therefore is a very effective immune booster.

Turmeric has long been used to treat the many symptoms of cold and flu along with bronchitis and sore throats.

In India, turmeric is used orally to treat gum disease and is also very effective when mixed with a dap of coconut or hemp oil and applied topically to a toothache.

Turmeric helps promote weight loss and lowers the incidences of obesity related diseases. The inflammation associated with weight increase is due in part to the presence of macrophages immune cells in fat tissues.

To get the most out of turmeric, add 3% black pepper to it. Black pepper improves the bioavailability of turmeric, which has the effect of making smaller quantities of turmeric more effective.

A 2008 study published in the journal *Drugs in R &D* found that a standardized preparation of curcuminoids made from turmeric compared favorably to the drug atorvastatin – trade name *Lipitor*. A human clinical study published in the journal *Diabetes Care* reveals that turmeric extract was 100% successful at preventing prediabetic patients from becoming diabetic.

A 1999 study published in the journal *Phytotherapy Research* found that the primary polyphenol in turmeric, the saffron colored pigment known as curcumin, compared favorably to steroids in the management of chronic anterior uveitis, an inflammatory eye disease.

Researchers at UCLA's *Jonsson Comprehensive Cancer Center* have shown that curcumin suppresses a cell signaling pathway that controls head and neck cancer growth. It has been shown that many of turmeric's medicinal value stems from its anti-inflammatory effects.

Effective as 14 Pharmaceutical Drugs

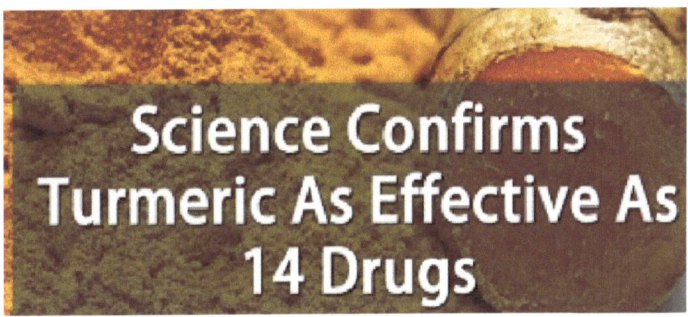

A number of published, peer-reviewed studies conducted over the years show turmeric as being the same as or better than 14 pharmaceutical drugs currently on the market including, but not limited to the following: (from GreenMedInfo.com):

1. Statin drugs for cholesterol- Lipitor (atorvastatin calcium) and Crestor (rosuvastatin)

2. Corticosteroid drugs – steroid medications used to treat arthritis and inflammatory eye disease

3. Antidepressants – Prozac and Paxil

4. Blood thinners – people at risk of heart attack or stroke

5. Anti-inflammatory drugs – ibuprofen, naproxen sodium and other pain pills

6. Chemotherapy drugs – Eloxatin; Oxaliplatin

7. Diabetes drug – Metformin (500-100,000 more effective)

Since turmeric helps to produce bile in the liver, turmeric is important in the detoxification process since bile production is essential in ridding the body of toxins. Bile carries accumulated toxins from the liver to the gallbladder then elimination in the feces completes this detoxification cycle.

Biopiracy

EXAMPLES OF BIO-PIRACY

1. US Patent 5401504 granted for the use of turmeric powder for healing wounds. Applicant did not disclose fully existence traditional knowledge on the subject matter in India. This was made available by India to USPTO, and the patent was revoked.

2. European Patent Office granted Patent EP0436257 on a method for controlling fungi on plants by the aid of a hydrophobic extracted neem oil, a knowledge that was extensively used in India already. NGOs and a European Parliament helped in getting the patent revoked.

In the mid 1990's, turmeric became subject to a patent dispute which had major global ramifications for international trade law. A U.S. patent on turmeric was awarded to the University of Mississippi Medical Center in 1995 specifically for "turmeric's use in wound healing". The patent granted the University the exclusive right to sell and distribute turmeric. Two years after this patent was granted, India's Council of Scientific and Industrial Research (CSIR) challenged the "novelty" of the University's "discovery" by filing a complaint. In India, where turmeric has been used for thousands of years, concerns grew about the economically damaging impact this patent could have on the legal biopiracy. CSIR located 32 references, some more than 100 years old, which showed that the "novel discovery" was well known in India prior to the patent application. The patent on turmeric was subsequently revoked in 1997.

Growing Turmeric

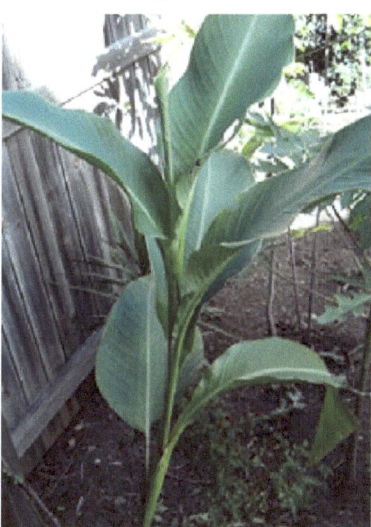

Turmeric in the garden

Turmeric can be cultivated for personal use by planting directly in the garden or in pots. Although turmeric is recommended for hardiness zones 9, it can be grown outdoor in the summer of colder zones too if placed in full sun whereas in hotter climates, turmeric can be placed where it will receive afternoon shade. When growing turmeric in a container, it is best to choose one that is at least 12 inches deep and equally as wide. Although turmeric can grow in almost any type of soil, it grows best in rich, well-drained soil, as clay soil will make it more difficult to care for. In hotter climates, turmeric requires lots of water.

Turmeric is grown from rhizomes or root cuttings, much like ginger, not from seed since turmeric does not propagate seeds. To plant, choose a small rhizomes or pieces with at least one or two buds and plant facing up, around two inches deep and sixteen inches apart to allow plenty of room to breathe and flourish. In zones 9-11, plant in the early fall and in northern growing zones, plant in the late spring, well after any chance of frost.

After the rhizomes are planted, it will usually take a few weeks for the root to sprout. Most herbs cab be harvested throughout the growing season, turmeric root is best if harvested all at once when it is fully mature usually after 7-9 months from planting. Signs that turmeric is fully mature and ready to harvest are when the bottom leaves of the plant have turned yellow.

After digging up the roots wash and clean and it is ready to use. Unpeeled roots can be stored in an airtight container and kept in a cool dark location for up to six months. If your preference is dried turmeric, then boil the roots for 45 minutes, peel and then let dry for about a week. Once dried, grind into fine orange or yellow powder and store in a cool dark place until ready to use.

Turmeric is dormant, even in hotter climates, in the winter months. Insects or diseases seldom bother turmeric. Aphids and mites may occasionally cluster on the leaves; they can be easily washed off with a spritz of water.

Turmeric Recipes for Beauty

The facial mask recipes that follow should be adjusted to suit individual preferences with the goal of reducing any possible waste

Turmeric helps cleanse the skin and maintain its elasticity; provide nourishment to the skin and balance the effects of skin flora.

Turmeric Lemon Juice Facial Mask

1 teaspoon turmeric powder

1 tablespoon of gram flour (chickpea, garbanzo bean or besan flour which can be found at an Indian grocery store)

A few drops of lemon juice

Milk

Instructions:

Mix the flour and turmeric together. Add the lemon juice and mix. Slowly add milk until a creamy paste is formed. Apply the mask to your clean face and neck. Leave the mask on for 15-20 minutes, until your skin feels tight and mask has dried. Wash the mask off using warm water and a washcloth. (Warning – the yellow pigment in turmeric will stain clothes. You may want to dedicate an older washcloth for your turmeric mask.

Result: glowing complexion

Turmeric Mask for Healing and Toning

Ingredients:

1 tsp. turmeric powder

1 tsp. sandalwood powder

¼ cup besan flour

1 tsp. almond oil

Instructions:

Combine dry ingredients. Add just enough oil to make a paste. Paint on face and neck and leave on for 20 minutes or until the mask dries. Wash the mask off using warm water and washcloth.

Benefits: Turmeric is used to counteract skin imbalances by reducing pimples and other spots on the face. Turmeric also hydrates the skin; adds color to pale skin and gives skin a radiant glow.

Turmeric & Coconut Oil Face Mask

By far the easiest turmeric mask to prepare and use. Simply mix a small dab of coconut oil with a enough turmeric powder to form a paste. Apply to face and neck in a circular motion and exfoliate for at least a couple of minutes. Leave the mask on for at least twenty minutes prior to washing off with warm water and a wash cloth.

Turmeric and Rice Powder Wrinkle Treatment

1 tsp turmeric powder

1 tsp rice powder (use a coffee grinder)

Raw milk

Tomato juice

Combine dry ingredients. Add just enough milk and tomato juice to make a face pack and apply to face and neck and leave on for 30 minutes. Wash the pack off using warm water and washcloth.

Turmeric and Lime Juice Face Whitening Paste

Mix one teaspoon of turmeric with three tablespoons of lime juice to form a thick paste. Apply evenly to the face or desired area. Wash off after fifteen minutes with warm water. Do not use soap as it will counteract the power of the paste. This paste can be used until desired results are achieved.

Turmeric for Whiter and Healthier Teeth

In a small dish or cup, combine turmeric powder with a small amount of water or coconut oil to make a paste. Scoop it up with the bristles of your toothbrush and brush like normal. Your toothbrush will be irreversibly colored yellow but your teeth will become whiter and stronger.

Turmeric Shake

Start your day by adding turmeric to your protein shake, green health drink or smoothie. Using either liquid turmeric or in powder form, it doesn't matter how it is added, just as long as it is added.

Anti-inflammatory Turmeric Tea

Ingredients:

32 oz. of boiling water

1 tablespoon turmeric powder

1 tablespoon of fresh ginger thinly sliced

1 handful of chopped cilantro

1 clove of garlic peeled and crushed

1 tablespoon of olive oil

2 lemons juiced

5 peppercorns whole

1 orange, juiced (or substitute 1 ½ tbsp. honey)

Instructions:

Boil water. Combine all ingredients in a strainer or teapot. Pour boiling water into the pot and steep for 10 minutes. Strain and enjoy.

Turmeric Tea for Cold and Flu

The following tea should be used with the onset of cold or flu symptoms to help fight bacterial infections and to reduce chronic inflammation.

4 cups of water

1 tablespoon ground turmeric

1 tablespoon of cinnamon

Black pepper

Lemon and honey are optional

Bring water to a boil, reduce heat, add turmeric and pepper and simmer for 10 minutes. Strain into a mug using a mesh strainer or cheesecloth. Add honey and/or lemon to taste

Soothing Turmeric Tea

1 cup of almond milk

1 teaspoon turmeric powder

½ tsp each of black pepper, cumin, cinnamon, cardamom, coriander

1 tsp honey or agave

Combine the above in a saucepan, heat slowly on low heat. Simmer for ten minutes; serve and enjoy.

Medicinal Turmeric Tea

1 cup of coconut milk

1 tsp each of turmeric and ginger powder

¼ tsp of Cayenne powder or according to taste

1 tsp honey

Blend the above in a saucepan; heat slowly on low and simmer for ten minutes. Serve and enjoy.

Other ways of enjoying turmeric:

Add turmeric to salad dressings; Turmeric is the perfect spice to use with lentils; Add turmeric to egg salads for a bolder color; Mix with onion and cottage cheese in the blender and serve as a dip with fresh vegetables

Mix brown rice with raisins and cashews and season with turmeric, cumin and coriander.

Turmeric Immune Boosting Soup

Ingredients:

1 tablespoon of coconut oil

1 chopped onion

1 head of garlic chopped

¼ cup chopped fresh ginger

2 tablespoons of turmeric powder

½ teaspoon of cayenne powder

4 cups of filtered water

1 teaspoon each of rosemary, cilantro, Himalayan salt and ground pepper

Choice of chopped vegetables such as carrots, celery, green beans

½ cup of barley, quinoa or rice

Instructions:

Roughly, chop onion, garlic, ginger and vegetables. Sauté chopped onion in coconut oil for three minutes then add chopped garlic and chopped ginger and continue to sauté for another three minutes. Add water followed by other ingredients and simmer for 20 minutes. Serve with hemp hearts or hemp flakes.

Vegetable Curry (serves 4)

Ingredients:

1-2 tablespoons coconut oil

1 medium onion, diced

2 cloves garlic, crushed

1 teaspoon curry powder

1 teaspoon cumin

½ teaspoon coriander

¼ teaspoon cinnamon

¼ teaspoon ground ginger

½ teaspoon turmeric

½ teaspoon Himalayan salt

½ butternut squash, peeled and cut into small cubes

¾ cup water

1 large sweet potato, peeled and cut into small cubes

½ head cauliflower, cut into small florets

¾ cup frozen organic peas

½ teaspoon garam masala

Cilantro (optional)

Instructions:

Sauté the onion and garlic in coconut oil until the onions are soft and opaque.

Add the spices, salt, pepper, and sauté a few minutes, until you can smell the aroma of the spices.

Stir the spices from the bottom of the pot occasionally.

Add the butternut squash and sauté about 10 minutes, stirring occasionally. Add 1 or 2 tablespoons of water to prevent sticking.

Add sweet potato and sauté about 10 minutes, stirring occasionally.

Add the rest of the water and scrape all the spices up from the bottom of the pot.

Add cauliflower and peas on top of the butternut and sweet potato, do not stir.

Cook until the vegetables are tender, about 10 – 15 minutes.

Just before serving, add garam masala and stir through.

Sprinkle with cilantro.

Veggie-Turmeric Quinoa

Ingredients:

1 tablespoons coconut oil

1 medium onion, diced

1 red bell pepper

2 cups cauliflower, cut into small pieces

Pink Himalayan salt and black pepper

1 Tbsp. curry

½ tsp turmeric

Cayenne pepper to taste

¾-cup dry quinoa

Instructions:

Bring 2 cups of water to a boil in a saucepan. Add quinoa, reduce heat, and simmer until the water is absorbed, about 15 minutes. Heat the coconut oil in a skillet pan and add the diced onions and lightly sauté for three minutes; add salt, curry, turmeric and black pepper. Add the other vegetables and lightly sauté for six minutes until soft yet not overcooked. Add the cooked quinoa, stir and serve.

Noteworthy

Important: Turmeric is fat-soluble and in order for our bodies to properly absorb the magnificent health benefits, turmeric should be consumed with a bit of fat such as coconut oil, hemp oil or olive oil. In addition, to further increase the effectiveness of turmeric, mix it together with a small amount of black pepper. Adding black pepper to turmeric enhanced food, can further enhance the bioavailability of turmeric by 1000 times.

Using turmeric can result in orange or yellow stains. To remove stains caused by turmeric on countertops, use baking soda with a little water and scrub the area, rinse and repeat the process as many times as necessary until the stain is gone. Alternatively, hydrogen peroxide can be used in all areas where turmeric has caused a stain to occur.

Conclusion

Turmeric has been used in Ayurveda Medicine and in Traditional Chinese Medicine for thousands of years for beauty, medicinal and many other household uses. Most turmeric in use is in the form of dried rhizome (root) powder. In some regions of India however, turmeric leaves are used to wrap and cook food as it offers a distinctive flavor in addition to health benefits. Turmeric's use as medicine has been used for thousands of years in the east and is only beginning to be recognized as a valuable medicinal source in North America.

The active compound curcumin is known to have a large range of biological effects including anti -inflammatory, antioxidant, anti-tumor, antibacterial, antiviral and antiseptic activities making it a valuable source of medicinal benefits for both internal and external use. As a secondary plant metabolite, its purpose is to enhance life.

If turmeric is not presently part of your beauty routine, the benefits derived are worth checking into.

.

About the Author

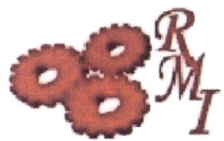

Ryder Management Inc.
Getting you in gear

Ryder Management Inc. (Rydermgt) is a Canadian Controlled Private Corporation (CCPC) based in London, ON Canada. As an "umbrella" organization, it brings together a group of authors whom are professionals in their respective fields and are writing with the primary goal of providing books that educate, comfort and offer assurance that natural remedies do exist and are an effective and safe way to enhance health.

The contributing author of our first book "*A Cancer Cure? The Amazing Health and Beauty Benefits of Turmeric*" was diagnosed with cancer and adamantly refused conventional cancer treatment used in Canada. Stephanie then began a quest for an alternative method of treatment that included online research, interviews and placing calls to India. This first book begins the series on herbal remedies that date back to ancient times. Included in this book are recipes using turmeric in a quantity sufficient to bring immediate results. Since discovering turmeric, the recipes are made/used regularly by Stephanie whereby she just won't stop talking about her findings. However, Turmeric really is nothing short of "amazing".